Managing Diabetes

A Comprehensive Guide to a Healthier Life

Rossana Lewis

TABLE OF CONTENT

Chapter 1: Understanding Diabetes

1.1 Defining Diabetes

Diabetes is a disease that occurs when your blood glucose, also called blood sugar, is too high. Glucose is your body's main source of energy. Your body can make glucose, but glucose also comes from the food you eat.

Insulin is a hormone made by the pancreas that helps glucose get into your cells to be used for energy. If you have diabetes, your body doesn't make enough or a any insulin, or doesn't use insulin properly. Glucose then stays in your blood and doesn't reach your cells.

Diabetes raises the risk for damage to the eyes, kidneys, nerves, and heart. It is also linked to some types of cancer. Taking steps to prevent or manage diabetes may lower your risk of developing diabetes health problems.

1.2 Types of Diabetes

The most common types of diabetes are type 1, type 2 and gestational diabetes.

Type 1 diabetes: If you have type 1 diabetes, your body makes little or no insulin. Your immune system attacks and destroys the cells in your pancreas that make insulin. Type 1 diabetes is usually diagnosed in children and young adults, although it can appear at any age. People with type 1 diabetes need to take insulin every day to stay alive.

Type 2 diabetes: If you have type 2 diabetes, the cells in your body don't use insulin properly. The pancreas may be making insulin but is not making enough insulin to keep your blood glucose level in the normal range. Type 2 diabetes is the most common type of diabetes. You are more likely to develop type 2 diabetes if you have risk factors, such as overweight or obesity, and a family history of the disease. You can develop type 2 diabetes at any age, even during childhood. You can help delay or prevent type 2 diabetes by knowing the risk factors and taking steps toward a healthier lifestyle such as losing weight or preventing weight gain.

Gestational diabetes: Gestational diabetes is a type of diabetes that develops during pregnancy. Most of the time, this type of diabetes goes away after the baby is born. However, if you've had gestational diabetes, you have a higher chance of developing type 2 diabetes later in life. Sometimes diabetes diagnosed during pregnancy is type 2 diabetes.

Prediabetes: People with prediabetes have blood glucose levels that are higher than normal but not high enough to be diagnosed with type 2 diabetes. If you have prediabetes, you have a higher risk of developing type 2 diabetes in the future. You also have a higher risk for heart disease than people with normal glucose levels.

A less common type of diabetes, called monogenic diabetes is caused by a change in a single gene. Diabetes can also come from having surgery to remove the pancreas or from damage to the pancreas due to conditions such as cystic fibrosis or pancreatitis.

1.3 Prevalence and Risk Factors

Diabetes is a global health issue of significant concern with its prevalence steadily rising across the world. Understanding the prevalence of diabetes is crucial to grasp the magnitude of this chronic condition's impact on individuals and societies. It is now considered an epidemic. According to data from the International Diabetes Federation (IDF), the number of people living with diabetes worldwide has been increasing at an alarming rate. In 2019, there were over 463 million adults diagnosed with diabetes and this number is projected to escalate to approximately 700 million by 2045. This statistic highlights the growing scale of the diabetes epidemic as it impacts one in every ten adults globally.

The vast majority of diabetes cases belong to Type 2 diabetes, which accounts for approximately 90% of all diabetes diagnoses. This form of diabetes is particularly prevalent in adults but it is increasingly being diagnosed in children and adolescents. The substantial rise in Type 2 diabetes cases can be directly linked to several factors, primarily lifestyle-related. While diabetes is a global concern, its prevalence varies from one region to another. Some areas, such as the Middle East, North America, and parts of Asia, have seen a more rapid increase in the prevalence of diabetes. Urbanization, changes in dietary habits, and reduced physical activity in these regions have contributed to the higher rates of diabetes.

Diabetes poses a substantial economic burden on healthcare systems and individuals. The costs associated with the treatment of diabetes and its complications are substantial. Moreover, the disease can lead to reduced productivity and, in severe cases, disability, which affects not only the individual with diabetes but also their families and communities.

Understanding the prevalence of diabetes is crucial for raising awareness and promoting proactive prevention and management strategies. Lifestyle modifications, such as adopting a healthy diet, engaging in regular physical activity, and maintaining a healthy body weight, play a pivotal role in preventing Type 2 diabetes. Routine medical check-ups, especially for those with risk factors, enable early diagnosis and timely intervention.

Additionally, addressing the societal determinants of health such as improving access to healthy food and promoting physical activity in communities, is essential in combating the diabetes epidemic.

In conclusion, the prevalence of diabetes is a pressing global health concern that demands attention, awareness, and action. By understanding the scale of the problem, individuals, healthcare professionals and policymakers can work together to implement strategies for prevention, early diagnosis, and effective management, ultimately reducing the impact of this chronic condition on individuals and societies.

Now let's look at the risk factors. For type 1 diabetes, it is thought to be caused by an immune reaction (the body attacks itself by mistake). Risk factors for type 1 diabetes are not as clear as for prediabetes and type 2 diabetes. Known risk factors include:

- Family history: Having a parent, brother, or sister with type 1 diabetes.
- Age: You can get type 1 diabetes at any age, but it usually develops in children, teens, or young adults.

In the United States, White people are more likely to develop type 1 diabetes than African American and Hispanic or Latino people. Currently, no one knows how to prevent type 1 diabetes.

For type 2 diabetes, you're at risk if you:

- Have prediabetes.
- Are overweight.

- Are 45 years or older.

- Have a parent, brother, or sister with type 2 diabetes.

- Are physically active less than 3 times a week.

- Have ever had gestational diabetes (diabetes during pregnancy) or given birth to a baby who weighed over 9 pounds.

- Are an African American, Hispanic or Latino, American Indian, or Alaska Native person. Some Pacific Islanders and Asian American people are also at higher risk.

If you have non-alcoholic fatty liver disease you may also be at risk for type 2 diabetes.

You can prevent or delay type 2 diabetes with proven lifestyle changes. These include losing weight if you're overweight, eating a healthy diet, and getting regular physical activity.

For prediabetes, you're at risk of you:

- Are overweight.

- Are 45 years or older.

- Have a parent, brother, or sister with type 2 diabetes.

- Are physically active less than 3 times a week.

- Have ever had gestational diabetes (diabetes during pregnancy) or given birth to a baby who weighed over 9 pounds.

- Are an African American, Hispanic or Latino, American Indian, or Alaska Native person. Some Pacific Islander and Asian American people are also at higher risk.

You can prevent or reverse prediabetes with proven lifestyle changes. These include losing weight if you're overweight, eating a healthy diet, and getting regular physical activity.

For gestational diabetes(diabetes while pregnant), if you:

- Had gestational diabetes during a previous pregnancy.
- Have given birth to a baby who weighed over 9 pounds.
- Are overweight.
- Are more than 25 years old.
- Have a family history of type 2 diabetes.
- Have a hormone disorder called polycystic ovary syndrome (PCOS).
- Are an African American, Hispanic or Latino, American Indian, Alaska Native,

Native Hawaiian, or Pacific Islander person.

Gestational diabetes usually goes away after you give birth, but increases your risk for type 2 diabetes. Your baby is more likely to have obesity as a child or teen, and to develop type 2 diabetes later in life.

Before you get pregnant, you may be able to prevent gestational diabetes with lifestyle changes. These include losing weight if you're overweight, eating a healthy diet, and getting regular physical activity.

1.4 The Impact of Diabetes on Health

Diabetes can impact many parts of your body, including heart, kidneys, eyes, feet, and legs. Various complications are possible the longer you live with the condition and if you have higher blood sugars over time. When you hear the word "diabetes," your first thought is likely about high blood sugar.

Blood sugar is an often-underestimated component of your health. When it's out of balance over a long period of time, it could develop into diabetes.

Diabetes affects your body's ability to produce or use insulin, a hormone that allows your body to turn glucose (sugar) into energy.

Here are what symptoms may occur to your body when diabetes develops:
- risk of stroke
- extreme thirst
- sweet smelling breath

- risk of heart disease

- fatigue and lack of energy

- pancreas malfunction

- excessive urination

- damaged blood vessels

- nerve damage

- foot problems

- dry, cracked skin

- ketoacidosis

- protein in the urine

- High blood pressure

- gastroparesis

- risk of infections

- cataracts and glaucoma

- visual disturbances

- loss of consciousness

Diabetes can be effectively managed when diagnosed early. However, when left untreated, it can lead to potential complications that include:

- kidney damage
- heart disease
- nerve damage
- stroke

Normally after you eat or drink, your body will break down sugars from your food and use them for energy in your cells. To accomplish this, your pancreas needs to produce a hormone called insulin. Insulin is what facilitates the process of pulling sugar from the blood and putting it in the cells for use, or energy.

If you have diabetes, your pancreas either produces too little insulin or none at all. The insulin can't be used effectively. This allows blood glucose levels to rise while the rest of your cells are deprived of much-needed energy. This can lead to a wide variety of problems affecting nearly every major body system.

Chapter 2: Diagnosis and Understanding Your Numbers

2.1 The Importance of Early Diagnosis

Diabetic care often focuses on treatment of the condition. While treatment is important, early detection increases the potential for effective changes early in the disease process. There are many reasons why earlier detection of diabetes could be of benefit to the individual and the health system, because it creates the opportunity to treat the high blood sugar and the risk factors for heart disease that often show up with diabetes. Individuals who don't know that anything is wrong may suffer long-term effects such as cardiovascular disease and stroke.

Furthermore, undiagnosed diabetes often results in potentially preventable, costly complications. Hospital stays could be avoided if patients are aware of their illness and work to manage it. Diabetes can be expensive. The estimated cost of living with diabetes is around $9,600 per year. This covers prescription medications, diabetic testing supplies, doctors appointments, and hospital care. Medical expenses rise drastically when emergency room visits are needed for unmanaged diabetic complications.

2.2 Blood Glucose Levels

Keeping your blood sugar in a target range reduces your risk of problems such as diabetic eye disease (retinopathy), kidney disease (nephropathy), and nerve disease (neuropathy). Some people can work toward lower numbers, and some people may need higher goals. For example, some children and adolescents with type 1 or type 2 diabetes, people who have severe complications from diabetes, people who may not live much longer, or people who have trouble recognizing the symptoms of low blood sugar may have a higher target range. And some people, such as those who are newly diagnosed with diabetes or who don't have any complications from diabetes, may do better with a lower target range.

Work with your doctor to set your own target blood sugar range. This will help you achieve the best control possible without having a high risk of hypoglycemia.

This is a suggestion for the following A1c and blood glucose ranges as general guide:

Most adults (non-pregnant)

- A1c: 7.0% or less
- Blood glucose:
  - Fasting and before meals: 4.0 to 7.0 millimoles per litre (mmol/L)
  - 2 hours after meals: 5.0 to 10.0 mmol/L or 5.0 to 8.0 mmol/L if A1c targets are not being met

Women with type 1 or type 2 diabetes who become pregnant

- A1c: 6.5% or less (6.1% or less if possible)
- Blood glucose:
  - Fasting and before meals: Less than 5.3 mmol/L
  - 1 hour after meals: Less than 7.8 mmol/L

- 2 hours after meals: Less than 6.7 mmol/L

Women with gestational diabetes

- Blood glucose:
    - Fasting and before meals: Less than 5.3 mmol/L
    - 1 hour after meals: Less than 7.8 mmol/L
    - 2 hours after meals: Less than 6.7 mmol/L

Children with type 1 diabetes (0 to 18 years old)

- A1c: 7.5% or less
- Blood glucose:
    - Fasting and before meals: 4.0 to 8.0 mmol/L

o 2 hours after meals: 5.0 to 10.0 mmol/L

Children, adolescents, and young adults with type 2 diabetes (up to 18 years old)

- A1c: 7.0% or less

2.3 HbA1c and its Significance

HbA1c test stands for glycated or glycosylated hemoglobin test. This test helps measure average blood sugar levels for the past 3 months. It is essential for every person who has diabetes. Other names of this test are glycohemoglobin test, A1c test, or simply A1c.

Hemoglobin is the protein in the red blood cells that help in transportation of oxygen across the body. Sugar (or glucose) present in the blood combines with one type of hemoglobin

(hemoglobin A), this combination molecule is called glycated hemoglobin. A red blood cell lives up to 120 days, or 4 months. Hence, measuring this combination molecule gives a fair estimate of your blood sugar levels in the last 2-3 months.

Do you regularly measure your fasting and after meal blood sugar to keep a check on your diabetes? Think that is enough? Not actually! Though the fasting and post meal tracking of blood glucose is important, these tests can only check your blood sugar at a certain point of time. Their results might vary depending on what you had eaten over the last night or in the previous meal. However, the HbA1c test looks at the 3-month data and cannot be biased. For persons having diabetes, HbA1c numbers give a fair idea of how controlled their diabetes is. As per scientific evidence, having a smaller HbA1c number means lesser risk of developing complications due to diabetes. All diabRaised HbA1c value has also been regarded as an independent risk factor for heart disease and stroke in people with or without diabetes.

The HbA1c test is used for diagnosis as well as monitoring purposes. Your doctor suggests an HbA1c test to see whether your diabetes is controlled or not. Pre-diabetics, people having borderline diabetes, are also advised to get tested to check how stable their blood sugar levels are. All diabetic patients should know the significance of the hba1c test.

2.4 Monitoring Your Blood Sugar

If you have diabetes, monitoring your blood sugar (glucose) is key to finding out how well your current treatment plan is working. It gives you information on how to manage your diabetes on a daily and sometimes even hourly basis.

Monitoring your blood sugar is important when you have diabetes, especially if you use insulin. The results of blood sugar monitoring can help you make decisions about food, physical activity and dosing insulin. Several things can affect your blood sugar. You can learn to predict some of these impacts with time and practice, while others are very difficult or impossible to predict. That's why it's important to check your blood sugar regularly if your healthcare provider recommends doing so. For example, the following situations typically raise blood sugar levels:

- Consuming carbohydrates.

- Not taking enough diabetes medication or insulin or missing a dose.
- Consistent lack of exercise or getting less activity than you usually do.
- Taking corticosteroid (steroid) medications.
- Illness, surgery or stress.
- Dawn phenomenon (an early-morning rise in blood sugar that's likely due to natural fluctuations in hormones, such as cortisol).
- Smoking.
- Dehydration.
- Puberty.

The following situations typically lower your blood sugar:

- Missing meals.

- Taking too much diabetes medication or insulin.
- Physical activity.

The following situations can raise and/or lower your blood sugar depending on other factors and your unique biology:

- Periods (menstruation).
- Food and medication/insulin timing.
- Drinking beverages containing alcohol.
- Non-diabetes medication interactions.

Due to all of these varying factors, it's essential to monitor your blood sugar if you have diabetes. It's the only way to know for sure when your blood sugar levels are changing. And it helps you and your healthcare provider know how to adjust your management.

Chapter 3: Types of Diabetes Management

3.1 Medications and Insulin

Managing diabetes often requires a multi-faceted approach and for many individuals, medications and insulin therapy play a vital role in achieving blood sugar control. Understanding the different medications and insulin options available is essential for effectively managing diabetes. There are different medications for insulin:

Oral Medications: These are medications taken in pill form and are primarily prescribed for people with Type 2 diabetes. They work in various ways, such as by increasing insulin sensitivity, reducing sugar production in the liver, or helping the pancreas release more insulin. Common oral medications include metformin, sulfonylureas, DPP-4 inhibitors, SGLT2 inhibitors, and GLP-1 receptor agonists.

Injectable Medications: In some cases, injectable medications, other than insulin, are prescribed for individuals with Type 2 diabetes who have difficulty managing their blood sugar with oral medications alone. These injections often include GLP-1 receptor agonists, which stimulate insulin release and reduce blood sugar levels.

Insulin: Insulin therapy is a mainstay for people with Type 1 diabetes and is also prescribed for many individuals with Type 2 diabetes, especially as the disease progresses. Insulin is a hormone that helps regulate blood sugar levels by allowing glucose to enter the body's cells.

There are different types of insulin, categorized by their onset, peak, and duration of action. There are different types of insulin:

- Rapid-Acting Insulin: This type of insulin starts working within 15 minutes and peaks within one to two hours. It's typically taken just before or after meals to manage post-meal blood sugar spikes.

- Short-Acting Insulin: Short-acting insulin begins working within 30 minutes and peaks between two to four hours after injection. It's taken before meals to manage blood sugar levels during and after eating.

- Intermediate-Acting Insulin: Intermediate-acting insulin has a slower onset, usually within two to four hours, and peaks within four to 12 hours. It's used to help maintain blood sugar levels between meals and overnight.

- Long-Acting Insulin: Long-acting insulin provides a slow, steady release of insulin and typically has no pronounced peak. It helps maintain baseline blood sugar levels throughout the day and night.

- Ultra-Long-Acting Insulin: This newer class of insulin provides an even more extended release, often lasting 24 hours or longer, allowing for once-daily dosing.

The choice of medication or insulin type, as well as the delivery method, should be personalized based on an individual's unique needs, lifestyle, and diabetes management goals. Working closely with a healthcare provider is crucial to finding the most effective treatment plan.

Managing diabetes through medication and insulin therapy, when necessary, is a crucial aspect of achieving blood sugar control. Regular monitoring, adherence to medication regimens, and a healthy lifestyle are key components of successful diabetes management. It's important to consult with a healthcare provider to determine the most appropriate treatment plan for your specific type and stage of diabetes.

3.2 Lifestyle Changes

Working closely with your doctor, you can manage your diabetes by focusing on six key changes in your daily life.

Eat Healthy: This is crucial when you have diabetes, because what you eat affects your blood sugar. No foods are strictly off-limits. Focus on eating only as much as your body needs. Get plenty of vegetables, fruits, and whole grains. Choose nonfat dairy and lean meats. Limit foods that are high in sugar and fat. Remember that carbohydrates turn into sugar, so watch your carb intake. Try to keep it about the same from meal to meal. This is even more important if you take insulin or drugs to control your blood sugars.

Exercise: If you're not active now, it's time to start. You don't have to join a gym and do cross-training. Just walk, ride a bike, or play active video games. Your goal should be 30 minutes of activity that makes you sweat and breathe a little harder most days of the week. An active lifestyle helps you control your diabetes by bringing down your blood sugar. It also lowers your chances of getting heart disease. Plus, it can help you lose extra pounds and ease stress.

Get Checkups: See your doctor at least twice a year. Diabetes raises your odds of heart disease. So learn your numbers: cholesterol, blood pressure, and A1c (average blood sugar over 3 months). Get a full eye exam every year. Visit a foot doctor to check for problems like foot ulcers and nerve damage.

Manage Stress: When you're stressed, your blood sugar levels go up. And when you're anxious, you may not manage your diabetes well. You may forget to exercise, eat right, or take your medicines. Find ways to relieve stress through deep breathing, yoga, or hobbies that relax you.

Stop Smoking: Diabetes makes you more likely to have health problems like heart disease, eye disease, stroke, kidney disease, blood vessel disease, nerve damage, and foot problems. If you smoke, your chance of getting these problems is even higher. Smoking also can make it harder to exercise. Talk with your doctor about ways to quit.

Watch Your Alcohol: It may be easier to control your blood sugar if you don't get too much beer, wine, and liquor. So if you choose to drink, don't overdo it. The American Diabetes Association says that women who drink alcohol should have no more than one drink a day and men should have no more than two. Alcohol can make your blood sugar go too high or too low. Check your blood sugar before you drink, and take steps to avoid low blood sugars. If you use insulin or take drugs for your diabetes, eat when you're drinking. Some drinks like wine coolers may be higher in carbs, so take this into account when you count carbs.

3.3 Dietary Management

Dietary management of Diabetes, nutrition and physical exercise, both have important roles to play for people who are living with diabetes. When combined with exercise, a healthy diet plan can help to keep your blood glucose levels within the range set by your health care professional. This will give you a better quality of life and reduce the need for diabetic medications or insulin.

What you eat and when you eat are critical factors to maintaining blood glucose levels. This usually means making changes to your diet by cutting out fatty and sugary foods and carefully monitoring your calorie intake. This doesn't sound like much fun, but diets for diabetes don't have to be boring.

With careful management, you can create a healthy diet plan which is both nutritious and tasty. And contrary to popular belief you don't have to completely cut out sugar or alcohol. You just have to cut down on your intake by eating smaller portions or enjoying them less often. So don't worry, you can still have the odd treat, now and then. The health benefits of dietary management for diabetes include:

- Helps to keep blood glucose level, blood pressure and cholesterol within the range set by your healthcare professional.

- Helps you reduce weight or maintain a healthy weight.

- Can delay or prevent the onset of complications caused by diabetes.

- Give you more energy, making you feel good for longer.

3.4 Exercise and Physical Activity

If you have diabetes, being active makes your body more sensitive to insulin (the hormone that allows cells in your body to use blood sugar for energy), which helps manage your diabetes. Physical activity also helps control blood sugar levels and lowers your risk of heart disease and nerve damage.

Getting atleast 150mins per week of moderate intensity physical exercise may just be a good startup for your diabetes management. One way to do this is to try to fit in at least 20 to 25 minutes of activity every day. Also, on 2 or more days a week, include activities that work all major muscle groups (legs, hips, back, abdomen, chest, shoulders, and arms). Examples of moderate-intensity physical activities include:

- Walking briskly
- Doing housework
- Mowing the lawn
- Dancing
- Swimming
- Bicycling
- Playing Sports

These activities work your large muscles, increase your heart rate, and make you breathe harder, which are important goals for fitness. Stretching helps to make you flexible and prevent soreness after being physically active.

3.5 Stress Management

Stress can cause some people to become ill. And when you have diabetes, stress can significantly affect your ability to control the disease. If you are under stress, you may skip meals or forget to take your medication, which will affect your blood sugar level. Although you can't completely remove stress from your life, there are several ways you can reduce it. And by learning to better manage stress, you can help keep your diabetes under control. Plus, with less stress, you can have the energy you need to eat right, exercise, and check your blood sugar.

Having ways to bust stress can also help you sleep better. That's great because when you don't get enough sleep, your blood sugar can rise.

Here are some tips:

Try to Have a Positive Attitude: When things seem to be going wrong, it's always easier to see the bad instead of the good. Find something good in each important area of your life: work, family, friends, and health. Thinking about the good can help you get through the bad times.

Be Nice to Yourself: What are your talents, abilities, and goals? Are you expecting too much from yourself? Don't expect more of yourself than you have or are able to give. It's OK to say "no" to things that you don't really want or need to do.

Accept What You Cannot Change

For those stressful situations or problems that cannot be changed, develop a simple plan of action. Ask yourself the following questions:

- "Will this be important 2 years from now?"
- "Do I have control over this situation?"
- "Can I change my situation?"

Talk to Someone About Your Stressors: Don't keep everything bottled up inside. If you don't want to talk with a family member or close friend, there are counselors and clergy trained to provide support and insight. Ask your doctor for recommendations if you would like to see a psychologist or counselor.

Exercise to Lower Stress: The benefits of exercise in reducing stress are well known. Exercise gives you a feeling of well-being and may relieve symptoms of stress. Think about what kinds of exercise help you relieve stress. You can blow off steam with hard exercise, recharge on a hike, or do a relaxing mind-body activity like yoga or tai chi. You'll feel better. Exercise doesn't just help you fight stress. It can lower your blood pressure and help you lose any extra pounds. Talk with your doctor before you start a new exercise program. Ask what type of exercise might be best for you.

Practice Relaxation Skills: Practice muscle relaxation, deep breathing, meditation, or visualization.

Chapter 4: Creating a Diabetes Management Plan

4.1 Setting Realistic Goals

Aside from the essential medical to-do list, you may want goals that will help you grow as a person. A healthy life is not only in terms of managing your diabetes, but is also to do with being an all-round healthy person: mentally, spiritually, and physically.

The following suggestions for goals are based around managing diabetes but they can lead to a new, more satisfying way of life. So, grab life by the horns and try one of these goals for diabetes self-management:

Find Friends With Diabetes: Not everyone quite understands what diabetes is or how it affects you. But another person with diabetes will know exactly what you're going through. It's inspiring to see how a friend manages the matters which you might otherwise have felt alone in dealing with. Your healthcare professional can be your first port of call, they might be able to set up a mentor for you or give tips on how to find local friends with diabetes. Alternatively, they could refer you to a mental healthcare professional such as a counsellor or therapist, if you feel like you need to talk to someone.

Try New Recipes, Cook Healthier Food: A healthy diet is beneficial for anyone, regardless of whether it's type 1 or type 2 diabetes. Take the opportunity to eat healthier by getting creative with your recipes. Find ingredients that make you passionate about what fuels your body.

Exercise: It's important for everyone. Every person needs 150 minutes of moderate-intensity physical activity 5 days a week. With diabetes, exercise helps with maintaining blood glucose levels and avoiding cardiovascular diseases.

Quit One of Your Vices: We all have our guilty pleasures. But if smoking is one of those, then it's vital to quit to improve diabetes control and general health. Smoking puts strain on the blood vessels (along with numerous additional hazardous effects on the body), a strain that those with diabetes don't need.

Or, maybe your vice is an infatuation with fast-food, or an over-consumption of coffee. Try quitting, and see how your body thanks you!

Take More Control: If you happen to feel like you're not in control, try looking at which areas you could feel more in control of. This is particularly the case for people who may have grown up with diabetes. Instead of letting your parent or loved one tell you when to check your blood glucose, have enough confidence in yourself to know that you can do it! Of course, everybody needs help, especially when it comes from those who care for your well-being. But it may feel empowering to take control of one small aspect that you didn't feel confident in before. Equally, if you feel overwhelmed, don't be afraid of talking about diabetes and a loved one for more help. The key is finding a balance.

Make Diabetes Management a Habit: Establishing a habit will mean diabetes management feel less of a chore and more like second nature. Making habits is hard, but after about a month of doing something even just a small thing – an action will start to stick! For those with insulin-dependent diabetes, splitting your bolus is a habit that can give more control over blood glucose. This method can be used if eating carbs or fatty food with a low glycemic index. It involves taking the first dose of insulin at the meal, and then another 2-4 hours later. Ask your healthcare professional for more advice. Testing blood glucose regularly is also an important habit. If you want to help your body, you can only be effective if you know what your body is doing. And if you want to know what your body has been responding to, get into the habit of making a log of your meals. As you probably know, there are numerous helpers out there to make recording meals smooth and easy.

Be Kind to Yourself: Pancreas, blood glucose meter, ketones, carbs, insulin. There's no two ways about it: diabetes means there is a great deal to think of. Even when you feel like you have everything under control, you can often end up being hard on yourself for not doing more. Instead, consider what you have accomplished each day and be proud of it. Focus on your strengths. Being kind to yourself is just as important as any other kind of self-care. In fact, taking a moment to reflect is helping yourself not only from a mental point of view, but from a physical one as well. With stress and diabetes, blood glucose increases so relax and treat yourself.

Do Whatever You Want: You're not defined by your diabetes. So, don't feel limited to goals for diabetes self-management. Go hang gliding, learn French, take up gardening etc.

4.2 Building a Support Network

Navigating the challenges of diabetes can be overwhelming but you don't have to face it alone. Building a support network is a crucial component of effectively managing this chronic condition. You could start building support with family and friends as they know you through and through. There will be no need to hide your identity and who you truly are. So your family and friends are people you could talk to help you cope.

Support groups are another way you could build your network. They provide a safe space to share experiences, advice, and concerns with others who have diabetes. These groups can be in-person or online, and they offer a sense of belonging and understanding that comes from connecting with individuals who are facing similar challenges.

Another is healthcare providers. Your diabetes care team, including your primary care physician, endocrinologist, and diabetes educator, are valuable sources of support and guidance. They can help you navigate your treatment plan, answer questions, and offer resources to aid in your diabetes management.

Online communities and resources, the digital age has made it easier than ever to connect with others dealing with diabetes. Online forums, social media groups, and reputable websites offer a wealth of information, support, and shared experiences.

4.3 Working With Healthcare Professionals

In the management of diabetes, healthcare professionals are your trusted partners on the journey to better health. Collaborating effectively with your healthcare team is essential for understanding your condition, optimizing your treatment plan, and achieving long-term well-being. Your diabetes care team is typically composed of various professionals, each contributing unique expertise to your overall management. It may include the following:

Primary Care Physician: Your primary care doctor often serves as the coordinator of your healthcare team. They can diagnose diabetes, provide initial treatment, and monitor your overall health.

Endocrinologist: An endocrinologist is a specialist in hormonal disorders, including diabetes. They are often involved in the management of complex diabetes cases.

Diabetes Educator: Certified diabetes educators are knowledgeable in diabetes management and can help you understand your treatment plan, provide guidance on blood sugar monitoring, and assist with medication or insulin management.

Dietitian/Nutritionist: A registered dietitian or nutritionist can help you create a personalized meal plan, make dietary adjustments, and manage your blood sugar through nutrition.

Pharmacist: Pharmacists can provide information on diabetes medications, including dosages, potential side effects, and drug interactions.

Podiatrist: Foot care is essential for people with diabetes, as nerve damage and circulation issues can lead to foot problems. A podiatrist specializes in foot care.

Ophthalmologist/Optometrist: Diabetes can affect your vision. Regular eye exams with these professionals help detect and manage diabetes-related eye issues.

Mental Health Professional: Diabetes management can take a toll on your mental health. Psychologists or counselors can help you cope with emotional challenges and stress related to your condition.

Working collaboratively with your healthcare team can yield several benefits such as understanding your diabetes condition, treatment strategies that best suit you and the ailment, track your health progress and addressing your mental wellbeing.

4.4 Personalized Diabetes Care Plan

Diabetic care planning is a process which aims to provide patients with more control over the management of their condition. Diabetes is a multifaceted condition that affects numerous body systems altering their function. As such, diabetic patients must attend regular appointments with a multidisciplinary team of doctors and health professionals to optimally manage their condition. As diabetes can affect everyone differently, these health professionals work with the patient to create and follow a diabetic care plan based on the patients' individual needs. Diabetic care plans are an integral component of successful, long-term diabetes management. Essential components of a diabetic care plan include:

- Diet and exercise plan
- Compliance to prescribed medications
- Scheduled appointments with health professionals (podiatrists, dietician, diabetes educators)
- Individual health goals
- Regular care plan appointments give the patient a chance to discuss set goals,

experiences, worries and results of diabetic checks.

Owing to the nature of this health condition, there are a number of lifestyle and dietary changes that are required to prevent complications. On a regular basis, patients must monitor their blood glucose levels, participate in physical activity, consume specific medications, and eat a healthy diet. Diabetic care plans assist patients in maintaining this schedule and provide greater control of their self-care.

Chapter 5: The Role of Diet in Diabetes Management

5.1 The Impact of Food on Blood Sugar

Whether you have recently been diagnosed with diabetes or prediabetes, or have been managing it for years, you probably know that what you eat has a big impact on your blood glucose. There's no set number of carbs that everyone with diabetes should eat. The eating plan and carb amount that works for you will depend on your gender, activity level, and blood glucose management plan, among other things. It will also depend on your current eating habits, food preferences, and budget.

Depending on your current eating habits, making some adjustments to your carb intake may help with blood glucose management. But, there's no need to make drastic changes to your diet all at once and you don't have to eat foods you don't like!

Consuming foods rich in carbohydrates, especially simple carbohydrates like sugar and white bread, can lead to rapid spikes in blood sugar. Complex carbohydrates, such as whole grains and vegetables have a slower and more controlled effect.

For proteins, they have minimal impact on blood sugar levels. They can cause a slight increase in blood sugar, but this effect is typically slower and less pronounced compared to carbohydrates.

Fats have a minimal and delayed impact on blood sugar. While they don't cause a rapid increase in blood sugar, high-fat meals can affect blood sugar levels hours after consumption.

Also, foods rich in dietary fiber, such as fruits, vegetables, and whole grains, can slow the absorption of sugar from other carbohydrates. This can help stabilize blood sugar levels and prevent rapid spikes.

It's important to recognize that individual responses to food can vary. What affects one person's blood sugar may not affect another's in the same way. Factors like genetics, insulin sensitivity, and overall health can influence individual responses to food.

5.2 The Basics of Carbohydrate Counting

Carb counting at its most basic level involves counting the number of grams of carbohydrate in a meal and matching that to your dose of insulin. If you take mealtime insulin, that means first accounting for each carbohydrate gram you eat and dosing mealtime insulin based on that count. You will use what's known as an insulin-to-carb ratio to calculate how much insulin you should take in order to manage your blood sugars after eating. This advanced form of carb counting is recommended for people on intensive insulin therapy by shots or pump, such as those with type 1 and some people with type 2.

While people with type 2 diabetes who don't take mealtime insulin may not need detailed carb counting to keep their blood sugars in line, some prefer to do it. While some choose to stick with traditional carb counting, there are others who do a more basic version of carb counting based on "carbohydrate choices," where one "choice" contains about 15 grams of carb. Still others use the Diabetic Plate Method to eat a reasonable portion of carb-containing foods at each meal by limiting whole grains, starchy vegetables, fruits or dairy to a quarter of the plate.

So, there are a few ways to go about it and it's really about personal preference, but remember that the best carb counting method for you is the one that addresses your medication and lifestyle needs. As for the ideal number of carbs per meal, there's no magic number. How much carbohydrate each person needs is in large part determined by your body size and activity level. Appetite and hunger also play a role.

5.3 The Glycemic Index

The glycemic index (GI) is a value used to measure how much specific foods increase blood sugar levels. Foods are classified as low, medium, or high glycemic foods and ranked on a scale of 0–100. The lower the GI of a specific food, the less it may affect your blood sugar levels.

Keep in mind that the glycemic index is different from the glycemic load (GL). Unlike the GI, which doesn't take into account the amount of food eaten, the GL factors in the number of carbs in a serving of a food to determine how it may affect blood sugar levels. For this reason, it's important to take both the glycemic index and glycemic load into consideration when selecting foods to help support healthy blood sugar levels.

Following a low glycemic diet may offer several health benefits, including:

Improved Blood Sugar Regulation: Many studies have found that following a low GI diet may reduce blood sugar levels and improve blood sugar management in people with type 2 diabetes

Increased Weight Loss: Some research shows that following a low GI diet may increase short-term weight loss. More studies are needed to determine how it affects long-term weight management.

Could Benefit People With Fatty Liver: A low-glycemic diet could help reduce liver fat and liver enzyme levels in people with non-alcoholic fatty liver disease.

5.4 Meal Planning and Portion Control

Controlling your portions doesn't mean you need to eat tiny amounts or measure out precisely the number of peas on your plate. But if we're eating too much, then we may need to retrain our brains to see a smaller-than-normal portion as satisfying enough. Here are some tricks to try:

Use a Smaller Plate: A standard-sized portion will look small on a larger plate, making you feel dissatisfied. Use a smaller plate to prevent overloading.

Don't Double Your Carbs: If you already have some starchy carbohydrate with your meal, do you need bread, naan or chapatis as well? You could be doubling your portion, so if you like to have some bread on the side, you'll need to cut down the amount of starchy carbohydrate on your plate accordingly.

Give Measuring Cups a Go: Finding it difficult to gauge the right amount to eat? Try using measuring cups. You don't need to have special cups, though; you could use any teacups, mugs or containers that work for you. It's just a simple way of measuring the amount for you every time.

Be Selective With Your Seconds: Finish your meal with fruit rather than chocolate cake. An apple will help to fill you up more than a couple of squares of chocolate, but both contain similar amounts of calories.

Don't Pick at Leftovers: Wasting food certainly isn't ideal but it doesn't mean you need to finish off everyone else's portions. Avoid the temptation to polish off children's or grandchildren's meals or to nibble leftovers when there's not quite enough for a whole portion. If you find it happens regularly, then get into the habit of cooking less or have a plan to use up leftovers in another meal.

20-Minute Rule: Think you haven't had enough? Wait for about 20 minutes before reaching for a second helping. It can take a little while for you to feel full after you have eaten. So avoid the temptation to keep eating and see if you get that feeling.

Check Food Labels: Make sure you know what portion the nutrition information on the front of pack relates to. It might be different to the amount you would normally serve yourself.

Ask For Less: When you're eating out, watch out for supersized portions. It's easier to avoid temptation if the food isn't on your plate to begin with, so say no to the bread basket and think about whether you need to have chips with your burger.

5.5 Managing Special Conditions and Dining Out

Going out to eat is a big part of our busy, modern lives. Although dining out can be super convenient (not to mention fun), many restaurants serve extremely large portions of high-calorie, high-fat, high-carbohydrate food.

These can be difficult to navigate when you need to maintain safe glucose levels.

Still, you don't have to miss out on the celebrations, events or even the just-don't-feel-like-cooking dinners that happen every day. There are ways to enjoy going out to eat while keeping your blood sugar at a healthy level. With your doctor's approval, give these tips a try:

Plan Ahead: Before going out to eat, be sure you have a general idea of what types of foods are available at the restaurant. Many places have menus online, and some have listed nutrition facts. Keeping in mind how many carbohydrates you can eat, look at the menu and pick out items that match your limits. If the restaurant does not list nutrition facts, scan the menu for lower-calorie preparation methods, such as steamed, grilled or broiled. Making your selection ahead of time helps you know you're making the best choice for your health when the server comes.

Choose the Right Beverage: Water and unsweetened tea are your best bets at a restaurant. That's because sugary beverages (juice and soda) cause your blood sugar to spike even faster than most foods. Some restaurants also offer free refills on soda without you asking. If it's front of you, you're more likely to drink it. If you want to drink alcohol, try to limit the quantity and avoid any sweet mixers — again, juice and soda.

3. Skip the Bread: Bread or chips regularly served before meals are high in carbohydrates —

and easy to eat mindlessly. It can be difficult to maintain normal glucose levels if you start your meal with a large dose of carbs. To help yourself out, ask the server to take the breadbasket away or not bring it at all.

Start Your Meal With Soup or Salad: A broth-based soup with loads of vegetables or a dinner salad is a great way to fill up on fiber with few calories or carbohydrates. Fiber is great if you have diabetes because it can help stabilize blood sugar. Stay away from high-calorie dressings, opting for olive oil and vinegar instead. Starting with a healthy soup or salad can help curb your hunger so you don't start your entree feeling starved, which can lead to overeating.

Swap the Sides: Restaurants often are glad to accommodate special requests, so feel free to swap out items on the menu. To keep your blood sugar steady, ask to substitute any high-carbohydrate sides — French fries, bread or potatoes with an extra serving of vegetables. This will save you a huge number of carbohydrates and calories and keep your blood glucose from spiking.

Take Home Half: Before your meal even begins, consider boxing up half right when it arrives to take home. You can also ask you server to box it before bringing it to the table, which is convenient and can save some temptation. You can also consider sharing an entrée with a friend. Considering portion sizes at many restaurants, these are great ways to cut calories and prevent overindulging.

Practice a Polite Response: Depending on who you are sharing a meal with, some people can try to derail your commitment to a diabetes-friendly diet. Do you have that friend who always wants dessert, but wants to share it? Or who says "just one bite won't hurt?" Be sure to have a plan ready for dealing with these types of situations. Brainstorm a polite response for these types of requests so you can be prepared. While you get the hang of adjusting your dining out habits, it's important to check your blood sugar levels after eating. Based on your readings, you can determine if you need to make more adjustments next time. Overall, you can eat healthfully and enjoy yourself with a bit of planning and a few intentional decisions.

Chapter 6: Exercise and Physical Activity

6.1 Benefits of Exercise for Diabetes

Like I said earlier in the previous chapter, being active makes your body more sensitive to insulin if you have diabetes which helps manage diabetes. Physical activity also helps control blood sugar levels and lowers your risk of heart disease and nerve damage.

Some of the benefits of exercise are:

- Usually lowers your blood sugar.

- Improves insulin sensitivity, which means your body's insulin works better. Note: You may need an adjustment in your diabetes medication or insulin dose to help prevent the blood sugar from going too low. Ask your health care provider for advice.

- Reduces body fat.
- Helps to build and tone muscles.
- Lowers your risk for heart disease.
- Improves circulation.
- Preserves bone mass.
- Reduces stress and enhances quality of life.

6.2 Types of Exercise

Exercise is good for pretty much everyone. It's especially important if you have diabetes. Workouts can do all kinds of things for you, like lower your blood sugar and blood pressure, boost your energy, and help you sleep better. If physical, high-impact exercises aren't for you, there are plenty of other options.

Walk: It's a simple way to get exercise and fresh air. It can lower your stress, too. A brisk stroll of 30 minutes to an hour 3 or 4 times a week is one way to hit your target. It's easy to get started. Take your dog around the neighborhood or walk to the store instead of driving. Once you've made it a habit, it can be rewarding and motivating to track your steps and your progress.

Dance: This can be a fun way to get your exercise. Just shake your groove thing for 25 minutes, 3 days a week to help your heart, lower your blood sugar, ease stress levels, and burn calories. You don't need a partner to get started, either. A chair can be good support if you need it.

Swim: This is one aerobic exercise that doesn't strain your joints like other ones can. It also lets you work muscles in your upper and lower body at the same time. Hitting the water is also good for your heart. It can also lower cholesterol and help you burn serious calories. If a lifeguard is on duty, let them know you have diabetes.

Bike: Fighting diabetes can be as easy as riding a bicycle. Whether you use a stationary one or hit the road, 30 minutes a day 3 to 5 times a week can get your heart rate up, burn blood sugar, and help you lose weight without hurting your knees or other joints.

Climb Stairs: This can be a healthy and easy way to burn calories and get your heart and lungs working faster, especially if you have type 2 diabetes. Going up and down stairs for 3 minutes about an hour or two after a meal is a good way to burn off blood sugar. You can do it anywhere there's a staircase, like when you need a break from work.

Strength Training: You do this with free weights or resistance bands. It can lower your blood sugar and help make your muscles and bones stronger. You get the most out of it if you do it twice a week in addition to your aerobic stuff. You can do many of these exercises at home like:

- Lifting canned goods or water bottles
- Push-ups
- Sit-ups
- Squats
- Lunges

Gardening: If the idea of traditional exercise isn't for you, don't worry. Time in your garden counts as both aerobic activity and strength training. It gets your blood going (since you're walking, kneeling, and bending). It also builds muscles and helps your bones (since you're digging, lifting, and raking). You're also outside, where your stress levels can be lower.

Yoga: It's worked for some 5,000 years as a low-impact exercise that can make you stronger and more flexible. Yoga can also help with balance. The motions, poses, and focus on breathing may also ease stress and help build muscle. That can keep your blood sugar levels more stable.

Tai Chi: This ancient Chinese art uses slow, controlled movements along with visualization and deep breathing to build strength. It can also help with mobility, balance, and flexibility. This gentle exercise can also lower your stress level. It may also help prevent nerve damage in your feet.

6.3 Overcoming Exercise Barriers

Everyone knows that exercise is good for you, but most people don't exercise. How do you move from knowing to doing? Take a good, honest look at why you are not exercising.

Time: Making time for physical activity during your week is key to creating a workout routine. Start by monitoring all your activities for a week and see where you can fit in three 30 min slots you could use for physical activity. If there aren't enough slots, try to find ways to add physical activity into your daily routine. Some examples of this include walking to work, climbing stairs or exercising while you watch TV. Also, while you are on the phone, try to stand, stretch or move as possible. This also works for watching movies. Another option is to add time into your schedule by waking up earlier in the morning.

Physical Pain or Fear of Injury: Pain or injury while exercising can be a holdup to resuming a workout routine or maintaining a current routine. Learning how to warm up and cool down will help prevent injury. When choosing a workout, consider your age, fitness level, and skill level. Don't start with heavy weightlifting if you haven't tried free weights. Start with activities you can do safely and increase the amount you do as your skills grow. Workout classes could be fun to try out new activities and find your favorites. In addition to weights and cardio exercises, balance, and flexibility activities are useful as well. As someone with diabetes, it is important to make sure your feet are in good shape. Check your feet daily for cuts, bruises, or sores. Make sure to see your foot doctor at least once a year. If your feet are numb or tingly, talk to your doctor before starting any physical activity.

Inconvenience: Whether it's time out of the day or motivation to go to the gym, adding exercise to your routine can be inconvenient at the beginning. Selecting activities you can do at home is a good way to start. Some examples of this include walking, jogging, or even investing in some inexpensive free weights for your home. There might also be resources within your community that you are able to take advantage of. Look for parks, recreation groups, and walking clubs to make friends and participate in activities close to home.

Lack of Motivation and Energy: To stay committed to an exercise routine, planning is critical. Without a plan, it is easy to take the path of least resistance, which is not participating in exercise. Scheduling physical activity for specific times or days in your calendar. That time is up to you, based on when you feel most energetic and what works with your schedule. Working with your nature and energy levels will lower the resistance to exercise. Additionally, set realistic expectations for incorporating exercise. Start with 1-2 times a week, and gradually increase as possible. A great way to stay committed to your exercise routine is to find support from friends and family. When beginning to exercise, explain to friends and family why you are doing this and ask for their support. Inviting your friends to participate in physical activity with you is a good way to socialize and improve your physical health at the same time! 1If your friends aren't up for it, finding additional friends to exercise with is possible. Join a local gym or walking club to find people with similar goals to offer support.

Boredom: Varying your fitness routine is helpful to avoid boredom. Finding various activities that you enjoy, such as weightlifting, or walking with friends. Changing between multiple activities that you enjoy will help avoid "falling into a rut" when it comes to exercise. Trying to be creative with increasing physical activity is key to overcoming barriers. Using these skills above will hopefully help you be successful in achieving your exercise goals.

6.4 Safety Precautions

Between work, school, and personal responsibilities, it can be challenging to add exercise to your routine. And if you have diabetes, you might worry that physical activity will lead to injury or make your condition worse. While these concerns are understandable, you shouldn't let them stop you from being active. There are steps you can take before you start a new routine and when you're exercising to avoid injury and other health problems. Below are few tips for exercising safely with diabetes:

Talk to Your Healthcare Provider Before Getting Started: Talk to your healthcare provider before you begin a new exercise program. This is a critical first step for people with Type 2 diabetes, because high blood glucose (hyperglycemia) can damage various organs and systems in the body.

Check Your Blood Glucose Before, During, and After Exercise If You Take Insulin: Insulin is a hormone that helps your body store and use the glucose that you get from food for energy. When you have Type 2 diabetes, your body isn't able to use insulin properly. As a result, your blood glucose levels rise over time and lead to health complications. Generally speaking, exercise can lower your blood glucose and help you manage your diabetes. But exercise also has the potential to make your blood glucose too low (hypoglycemia). So it's important to know how your body responds to physical activity.

Know your numbers: Talk to your healthcare provider about your own target blood glucose range as it may differ depending on your age and other factors. Knowing these numbers can help you stay in a safe range while exercising.

Fuel Yourself For Workouts and Replenish Afterward: A healthy diet can also help keep your blood glucose in a safe range during exercise. The best way to fuel your body depends on several factors, including your treatment plan, fitness goals, and the type of exercise you're doing.

Stay Hydrated: Everyone needs to properly hydrate in order to have safe and effective workouts. When you don't get enough fluids, it can lead to fatigue and poor exercise performance.

Find the Right Time: Research suggests that morning, afternoon, and evening workouts may affect your body differently. One very small study found that afternoon exercise helped men with Type 2 diabetes manage their blood glucose better than morning exercise, which increased blood glucose. But other experts suggest that morning workouts might be a good option for people who struggle with early-morning glucose spikes. The best time for you to exercise will depend on various factors, including your treatment regimen and schedule. Talk to your provider about ideal exercise times and monitor how your body responds to physical activity throughout the day. Once you find what works best for you, try to stay consistent by working out at the same time every day.

Check Your Feet: When you have nerve damage (diabetic neuropathy) in your feet, it may be harder to feel pain. So remember to check your feet for cuts, blisters, or other changes after every workout. When you exercise, wear supportive shoes to avoid injury. And if you have foot pain, consider activities that are easier on your feet, such as water aerobics, cycling, or chair yoga. Check in with your healthcare provider for regular foot exams and other tips to keep your feet healthy.

Listen to Your Body: Always listen to your body. A new exercise regimen may cause slight discomfort at first. But it shouldn't hurt. Stop your workout immediately if you notice new or concerning symptoms

Chapter 7: Monitoring Your Health

7.1 HbA1c Testing

Hemoglobin A1c, often referred to as HbA1c is a crucial test for individuals with diabetes. It provides a long-term perspective on blood sugar control, offering a comprehensive view of your average blood sugar levels over the past two to three months.

HbA1c works in a sense that in the form of hemoglobin, protein in red blood cells carry oxygen. When blood sugar (glucose) is in the bloodstream, it binds to hemoglobin. The amount of glucose bound to hemoglobin is directly related to the average blood sugar levels over the lifespan of red blood cells, which is typically two to three months. HbA1c testing measures the percentage of hemoglobin that has glucose attached to it. The result is presented as a percentage, and it indicates the average blood sugar level over the preceding two to three months.

HbA1c testing offers several key advantages for individuals with diabetes:

- Long-Term Monitoring: Unlike daily blood sugar measurements, which provide a snapshot of your current levels, HbA1c reflects your blood sugar control over an extended period. This comprehensive view helps identify trends and patterns that may not be evident from day-to-day measurements.

- Treatment Adjustment: HbA1c results guide healthcare providers in adjusting treatment plans. If your HbA1c level is consistently high, it may indicate a need for changes in medication, diet, or exercise.

- Goal Setting: HbA1c levels help set blood sugar control goals. Healthcare providers often work with patients to establish target HbA1c levels based on individual circumstances, such as age, overall health, and the presence of other medical conditions.

- Risk Assessment: High HbA1c levels are associated with a higher risk of diabetes-related complications, such as cardiovascular disease, kidney disease, and neuropathy. Monitoring HbA1c can help assess and mitigate these risks.

Now, how do you interpret HbA1c results set by the American Diabetes Association(ADA):

- Less than 5.7%: This is considered a normal or non-diabetic range.
- 5.7% to 6.4%: This range indicates prediabetes, which means a higher risk of developing diabetes.
- 6.5% or higher: An HbA1c level of 6.5% or above is typically used to diagnose diabetes.

For individuals with diagnosed diabetes, target HbA1c levels may vary, but the ADA generally suggests a target of less than 7% for most adults.

7.2 Blood Pressure and Cholesterol Control

Diabetes and high cholesterol may often occur together. High blood sugar and cholesterol levels increase the risk for stroke and heart attack. But, a healthy diet and lifestyle can help you control these. If you've been diagnosed with diabetes, you know that controlling your blood sugar levels is important. The more you can keep these levels down, the lower your risk of developing cardiovascular disease and other health problems.

Having diabetes puts you at a higher risk for developing high cholesterol. As you watch your blood sugar numbers, too. The main goal is to reduce your risk of heart disease and stroke. If you follow these seven tips, you'll be giving your body what it needs to stay healthy and active.

Watch Your Numbers: You already know that it's important to watch your blood sugar levels. It's time to watch your cholesterol numbers, as well. As mentioned previously, an LDL cholesterol level of 100 or less is ideal. Follow your doctor's instructions on keeping your blood sugar levels under control. Be sure to check on your other numbers during your annual doctor visits. These include your triglycerides and blood pressure levels. A healthy blood pressure is 120/80 mmHg. Those with diabetes shoot for a blood pressure of less than 130/80 mmHg. Total triglycerides should be less than 200 mg/dL.

Follow Standard Health Advice: There are some well-known lifestyle choices that clearly reduce the risk of cardiovascular disease. You probably know all of these, but just be sure that you're doing everything you can to follow them:

- Quit smoking or don't start smoking.
- Take all your medications as directed.
- Maintain a healthy weight, or lose weight if you need to.

After a Meal, Take a Walk: As someone with diabetes, you already know that exercise is key for keeping your blood sugar levels under control. Exercise is also key for managing high cholesterol. It can help increase levels of HDL cholesterol, which are protective against heart disease. In some cases, it can also reduce levels of LDL cholesterol. Probably the most effective exercise you can do to help control blood sugar levels is to take a walk after eating a meal.

Breathe a Little Harder Five Times a Week: In addition to walking after meals, it's also important to do some aerobic exercise for about 30 minutes daily five times a week.

Lift a Few Heavy Things: As we age, we naturally lose muscle tone. That's not good for our overall health, or for our cardiovascular health. You can resist that change by adding some weight training to your weekly schedule.

Plan Healthy Meals: You've probably already made changes in your diet to help keep your blood sugar levels low. You're controlling the amount of carbs you eat at each meal, choosing foods low on the glycemic index, and eating small meals more regularly. If you also have high cholesterol, this diet will still work for you, with just a few small modifications. Continue to limit unhealthy fats such as those in red meat and full-fat dairy, and choose more heart-friendly fats like those found in lean meats, nuts, fish, olive oil, avocadoes, and flax seed. Then simply add more fiber to your diet.

7.3 Eye and Dental Health

Diabetes can have detrimental effects on eyesight if not controlled. In fact, diabetes is the third leading cause of blindness in the United States. For this reason, it is recommended that everyone with diabetes see an ophthalmologist or an optometrist once a year for a dilated eye exam. But why? High blood glucose (aka blood sugar) can cause multiple complications in the eye. One example is Retinopathy, which is defined as damage to the retina in the eye that can cause impairment or loss of vision.

Retinopathy is the most common cause of vision loss in people with diabetes.

High blood glucose can also lead to cataracts and glaucoma. Most of the time an ophthalmologist or optometrist can detect these issues in the early stages and sometimes before vision is lost. If detected early, there are treatment options that may prevent blindness. It is also important to take care of your teeth. It has been said many times that the health of your teeth and gums can be a window to your overall health. Diabetes can have a great impact on oral health. Uncontrolled blood glucose can increase your risk for gum diseases such as gingivitis and periodontitis, cavities, and even tooth loss. But that may not be the only reason to brush and floss your teeth. There is some evidence that suggests that people with severe gum disease may have a harder time controlling their blood glucose, leading to worsening diabetes.

So what can you do to protect your eyes and teeth?

- Control your blood glucose. Most complications associated with diabetes stem from high levels of blood glucose over a period of time.
- Stop smoking or using tobacco. Tobacco use increases the risk for gum disease and blindness from retinopathy.
- Go to your regular check-ups. You should see the dentist every 6 months for a cleaning and dental exam and the ophthalmologist or optometrist at least once a year for a dilated eye exam.

- Maintain normal blood pressure. High blood pressure can increase your risk of retinopathy.

- Brush your teeth twice daily and floss every day to prevent cavities and gum infections.

7.4 Foot Care

Taking care of your feet when you have diabetes is an important part of your self-care regimen. Diabetic nerve damage can lessen your ability to feel sensations like pain, heat, and cold. This means that you may not even realize that you have a foot injury like a cut or blister until it gets infected. Nerve damage can even cause the shape of your feet and toes to change, making regular shoes uncomfortable and possibly damaging to your feet. Diabetes also causes blood vessels to narrow and harden, resulting in poor circulation (blood flow)—another culprit when it comes to foot complications. Poor circulation makes it more difficult for your foot to fight infection and heal. While even small cuts and ulcers can lead to more serious infections that result in loss of a limb, there are things you can do to protect your feet. Follow these tips to help prevent injury and reduce the risk of developing foot problems that can occur when you're living with diabetes and neuropathy.

Practice Good Daily Foot Care: Wash your feet well every day but refrain from using hot water. Instead, use warm soapy water and be sure to check your feet for sores, cuts, blisters, corns, or redness. Dry your feet carefully and apply a gentle moisturizer. Take care to avoid moisturizing between your toes which can lead to infections.

Trim Your Toenails: Keep toenails trimmed because long or thick nails can press on neighboring toes and cause open sores. Be sure to trim toenails straight across—cutting into the corners of nail can cause ingrown toenails. Finish by using an emery board to file down any sharp edges.

Choose the Right Footwear: Avoid going barefoot, even in your home, to reduce the risk of injury. Wearing socks and shoes (or slippers at home) gives feet extra protection. Plus, moisture-wicking socks help keep your feet clean and dry. Before putting your shoes on, check for any sharp objects like small rocks and wear shoes that fit properly without pinching your toes or rubbing against your feet. If your shoes aren't comfortable, ask your doctor about special therapeutic shoes or inserts that may be right for you.

Get Moving: Exercise is good for poor circulation. It stimulates blood flow in the legs and feet. Walk in sturdy, comfortable shoes that fit comfortably, but don't walk when you have open sores on your feet.

Work With Your Diabetes Care Team: Care for your feet and your overall health by controlling some of the things that cause neuropathy and poor blood flow. Follow your diabetes care team's advice for quitting smoking and keeping your blood glucose (blood sugar), blood pressure, and cholesterol under control. If you notice problems like numbness, ulcers, or cuts that have not healed, contact your doctor right away.

Chapter 8: Coping with the Emotional Aspects of Diabetes

8.1 The Psychological Impact of Diabetes

Depression is a medical illness that causes feelings of sadness and often a loss of interest in activities you used to enjoy. It can get in the way of how well you function at work and home, including taking care of your diabetes. When you aren't able to manage your diabetes well, your risk goes up for diabetes complications like heart disease and nerve damage. People with diabetes are 2 to 3 times more likely to have depression than people without diabetes. Only 25% to 50% of people with diabetes who have depression get diagnosed and treated. But treatment—therapy, medicine, or both—is usually very effective. And without treatment, depression often gets worse, not better.

Symptoms of depression can be mild to severe, and include:

- Feeling sad or empty
- Losing interest in favorite activities
- Overeating or not wanting to eat at all
- Not being able to sleep or sleeping too much
- Having trouble concentrating or making decisions
- Feeling very tired
- Feeling hopeless, irritable, anxious, or guilty
- Having aches or pains, headaches, cramps, or digestive problems
- Having thoughts of suicide or death

If you think you might have depression, get in touch with your doctor right away for help getting treatment. The earlier depression is treated, the better for you, your quality of life, and your diabetes.

8.2 Building Emotional Resilience

Emotional resilience is the ability to adapt and cope with adversity, stress, and life's challenges in a healthy and productive way. Living with diabetes can be a challenging journey that often requires significant emotional resilience. Managing a chronic condition, coping with daily self-care tasks, and facing potential complications can all take a toll on your emotional well-being. For individuals with diabetes, emotional resilience is crucial for several reasons:

Coping with Daily Management: Diabetes management involves daily tasks such as monitoring blood sugar levels, taking medications or insulin, and making dietary choices. These tasks can be emotionally taxing and require resilience to maintain consistency.

Dealing with Diabetes-Related Stress: Living with diabetes can lead to stress related to blood sugar fluctuations, medication management, and the fear of complications. Emotional resilience is essential for managing this stress effectively.

Preventing Burnout: Diabetes self-care is a lifelong commitment. Without emotional resilience, the burden of managing diabetes can lead to burnout, affecting your overall well-being.

Strategies for Building Emotional Resilience:

Education and Knowledge: Understanding diabetes, its management, and the potential complications can empower you with knowledge. Education can reduce the fear and anxiety often associated with the condition.

Support Network: Lean on family, friends, or support groups for emotional support. Sharing your feelings, challenges, and successes with others who understand can be immensely therapeutic.

Mindfulness and Stress Reduction: Mindfulness practices, such as meditation and deep breathing, can help reduce stress and improve emotional resilience. These techniques encourage living in the present moment and managing stress more effectively.

Regular Physical Activity: Exercise not only benefits physical health but also releases endorphins, which are natural mood elevators. Regular physical activity can reduce stress and improve emotional well-being.

Seek Professional Help: If you find yourself overwhelmed, anxious, or depressed due to diabetes, don't hesitate to seek help from a mental health professional. They can provide strategies to cope with emotional challenges and improve your quality of life.

Set Realistic Goals: Manage your expectations when it comes to diabetes management. Setting achievable goals can help prevent feelings of failure or frustration.

Maintain a Positive Outlook: Focus on the positive aspects of your life and health. Celebrate your successes, no matter how small, and practice gratitude.

Social Support: Interacting with friends and family who understand your diabetes management can be a source of emotional strength. Discuss your concerns, and let them be part of your support system.

Self-Care: Make time for self-care activities that you enjoy, such as reading, hobbies, or spending time in nature. These activities can help reduce stress and build emotional resilience.

Adaptive Problem-Solving: Instead of dwelling on setbacks, use adaptive problem-solving to find solutions to challenges in your diabetes management.

8.3 Seeking Support

Diabetes can seem overwhelming at times, but you can take control back. It helps to have people who encourage you and show you new ways to manage your diabetes day to day. Put them on your go-to list, and reach out any time you need their insight and motivation. Below are what you have to do to seek support:

See Your Specialists: You need a medical team that knows diabetes inside and out. They could include:

- An endocrinologist, who has a lot of experience working with people who have diabetes
- An ophthalmologist for your eyes
- A pharmacist, who's familiar with all your medicines
- A registered dietitian, who can give you pointers on what to eat
- A diabetes educator

All of these professionals work with you to help you stay well.

Join a Diabetes Support Group: It helps to talk to someone who can relate to what you're going through, since they have diabetes, too.

While support groups are not psychotherapy groups, they can provide you with a safe, accepting place to share your situation and get comfort and encouragement.

Include Your Friends and Family: Type 2 diabetes can affect the entire family. So get them, and your friends, involved. Share with them what you're going through and how you manage your diabetes. For instance, tell them why you have to check your blood sugar regularly, or what sorts of snacks and meals are OK for you. Want someone to help you get them up to speed? You might want to hold a family meeting, and invite your diabetes educator to answer their questions.

Consider Therapy: You deserve to feel good emotionally. If you don't, you may want to talk to a therapist. In therapy, you'll plan positive ways to handle your diabetes. It's not just for people with conditions like depression or anxiety. Anyone can benefit. You can get a fresh point of view that helps you work through your challenges. That's important, because stress can affect your blood sugar levels. Look for a licensed mental health professional who works with people who have diabetes or other long-term conditions. Ask your doctor for referrals. Pick someone you find easy to talk to. You might meet with your counselor one on one, with family members, or in a support group.

Chapter 9: Complications and Risk Reduction

9.1 Cardiovascular Health

Having diabetes means you are more likely to develop heart disease. People with diabetes are also more likely to have certain risk factors, such as high blood pressure or high cholesterol, that increase their chances of having a heart attack or a stroke. If you have diabetes, you can protect your heart and health by managing your blood glucose, also called blood sugar. You can also protect yourself by controlling your high blood pressure and high cholesterol. If you smoke, get help to stop.

High blood glucose from diabetes can damage your blood vessels and the nerves that control your heart and blood vessels. Over time, this damage can lead to heart disease. People with diabetes tend to develop heart disease at a younger age than people without diabetes. Adults with diabetes are nearly twice as likely to have heart disease or stroke as adults without diabetes. The good news is that the steps you take to manage your diabetes also help lower your chances of having heart disease or stroke.

Your risk for heart disease is greater if you are male rather than female, whether you have diabetes or not. If you do have diabetes, other factors add to your chances of developing heart disease or having a stroke such as

Smoking: Smoking raises your risk of developing heart disease. If you have diabetes, it is important to stop smoking, because both smoking and diabetes narrow blood vessels. Smoking also increases your chances of developing other long-term problems such as

- lung disease
- lower leg infections and ulcers
- foot or leg amputation

High Blood pressure: If you have high blood pressure your heart works harder to pump blood. High blood pressure can strain your heart, damage blood vessels, and increase your risk of heart attack, stroke, and eye or kidney problems. Have your blood pressure checked regularly and work with your doctor to control or lower high blood pressure.

Abnormal Cholesterol Levels: Cholesterol is a type of fat, produced by your liver and found in your blood. You have two kinds of cholesterol in your blood: LDL and HDL. LDL, often called "bad" cholesterol, can build up and clog your blood vessels. High levels of LDL cholesterol raise your risk of developing heart disease. HDL is sometimes called "good cholesterol." Higher levels of HDL is linked to lower risk for heart disease and stroke. To improve LDL and HDL levels, limit the amount of fat in your eating plan, eat more plant-based foods, and get regular physical activity. Another type of blood fat, triglycerides, also can raise your risk of heart disease when the levels are higher than recommended by your health care team.

Obesity and Belly Fat: Being overweight or having obesity can make it harder to manage your diabetes and raise your risk for many health problems, including heart disease and high blood pressure. If you are overweight, a healthy eating plan with fewer calories and more physical activity often will lower your blood glucose levels and reduce your need for medicines.

Excess belly fat around your waist, even if you are not overweight, can raise your chances of developing heart disease.

Family History of Heart Disease: A family history of heart disease may add to your chances of developing the condition. If one or more of your family members had a heart attack before age 50, you have double the chance of developing heart disease compared with people who have no family history of the disease. You can't change whether heart disease runs in your family. But if you have diabetes, it's even more important to take steps to protect yourself from heart disease and decrease your chances of having a stroke.

9.2 Kidney Health

Kidney health is a critical aspect of diabetes management. Diabetes is a leading cause of chronic kidney disease (CKD), and individuals with diabetes are at an increased risk of kidney-related complications. Understanding and proactively managing kidney health is essential for individuals with diabetes to prevent kidney problems and maintain overall well-being. Diabetes can have a profound impact on the kidneys due to the role these organs play in regulating blood sugar and filtering waste products from the body. The connection between diabetes and kidney health is as follows:

Glomerular Filtration: Diabetes can damage the glomeruli, which are tiny filters in the kidneys responsible for removing waste from the blood.

This damage can lead to a condition called diabetic nephropathy.

Microalbuminuria: A key indicator of early kidney damage in diabetes is the presence of small amounts of a protein called albumin in the urine, known as microalbuminuria. This condition can progress to more severe kidney problems if left uncontrolled.

Hypertension: High blood pressure (hypertension) often accompanies diabetes. Hypertension can further strain the kidneys, leading to kidney damage over time.

Strategies for kidney health risk reduction:
Blood Sugar Control: Maintaining stable blood sugar levels is paramount in preventing kidney damage. Regular monitoring and adherence to a

diabetes management plan can help control blood sugar and reduce the risk of kidney complications.

Blood Pressure Control: Managing blood pressure is equally crucial. Individuals with diabetes should work with their healthcare providers to maintain blood pressure within a healthy range.

Medication Adherence: Take prescribed medications as directed by your healthcare provider. Medications such as ACE inhibitors or ARBs are often used to protect kidney health in individuals with diabetes.

Healthy Diet: A diet low in salt, saturated fats, and processed foods can help manage blood pressure and reduce the risk of kidney damage.

Incorporate plenty of fruits, vegetables, whole grains, and lean proteins into your diet.

Hydration: Staying well-hydrated is essential for kidney health. Drinking an adequate amount of water can help your kidneys function optimally.

Quit Smoking: Smoking can exacerbate kidney damage. Quitting smoking is a positive step toward protecting your kidneys and overall health.

Regular Exercise: Physical activity can help control blood sugar and blood pressure, benefiting both diabetes and kidney health.

Regular Check-ups: Regular kidney function tests, such as estimated glomerular filtration rate (eGFR) and urinary albumin excretion, should be a part of your diabetes management plan. These tests can detect early kidney damage.

Educate Yourself: Understand the risk factors, symptoms, and complications of kidney disease. Knowledge is a powerful tool in proactive kidney health management.

9.3 Nerve Damage

High blood sugar can lead to nerve damage called diabetic neuropathy. You can prevent it or slow its progress by keeping your blood sugar as close to your target range as possible and maintaining a healthy lifestyle. Managing your blood sugar is an essential part of your diabetes care plan. Not only does it help you with day-to-day wellness, it can help prevent serious health problems down the road.

Nerve damage is one possible complication from having high blood sugar levels for a long time. High blood sugar damages your nerves, and these nerves may stop sending messages to different parts of your body. Nerve damage can cause health problems ranging from mild numbness to pain that makes it hard to do normal activities. Half of all people with diabetes have nerve damage. The good news is that you can help prevent or delay it by keeping your blood sugar as close to your target levels as possible. When you do this, you'll also have more energy, and you'll feel better!

Symptoms of nerve damage usually develop slowly, so it's important to notice your symptoms early so you can take action to prevent it from getting more serious.

There are different types of nerve damage: peripheral, autonomic, proximal and focal nerve damage. Keeping your blood sugar as close to your target range as possible is the best way to help prevent or delay nerve damage. Other things you can do are:

- Keep your blood pressure below 140/90 mm Hg (or the target your doctor sets).
- Get regular physical activity.
- Lose weight if you're overweight.
- Limit or avoid alcohol.
- Stop smoking or don't start.
- Follow a healthy eating plan.
- Take medicines as prescribed by your doctor.

9.4 Eye and Vision Health

Diabetes can damage your eyes over time and cause vision loss, even blindness. The good news is managing your diabetes and getting regular eye exams can help prevent vision problems and stop them from getting worse. Eye diseases that can affect people with diabetes include diabetic retinopathy, macular edema (which usually develops along with diabetic retinopathy), cataracts, and glaucoma. All can lead to vision loss, but early diagnosis and treatment can go a long way toward protecting your eyesight.

Diabetic Retinopathy is the leading cause of blindness in working-age adults. It is caused when high blood sugar damages blood vessels in the retina (a light-sensitive layer of cells in the back of the eye). Damaged blood vessels can swell and leak, causing blurry vision or stopping blood flow. Sometimes new blood vessels grow, but they aren't normal and can cause further vision problems. Diabetic retinopathy usually affects both eyes. Anyone with type 1, type 2, or gestational diabetes (diabetes while pregnant) can develop diabetic retinopathy. The longer you have diabetes, the more likely you are to develop it. These factors can also increase your risk:

- Blood sugar, blood pressure, and cholesterol levels that are too high.
- Smoking.
- Race/ethnicity: African Americans, Hispanics/Latinos, and American Indians/Alaska Natives are at higher risk.

Chapter 10: Living Well With Diabetes

10.1 Integrating Diabetes Management in your Life

Living with diabetes is a lifelong journey that involves daily self-care and management. It's important to find ways to seamlessly integrate diabetes management into your daily life to ensure that you can effectively control your blood sugar levels and prevent complications. To make diabetes management a natural part of your routine, here are some strategies:

Education and Knowledge: Understanding your condition is the first step to effective diabetes management. Learn about the different types of diabetes, the role of insulin, the impact of diet and exercise, and how to monitor your blood sugar levels. Knowledge empowers you to make informed decisions.

Create a Support Network: Share your diabetes journey with family and friends. They can provide emotional support and help you stick to your management plan. Consider joining diabetes support groups, both in-person and online, to connect with others who understand your challenges.

Meal Planning and Nutrition: Plan your meals and snacks in advance to ensure you make healthy food choices. Incorporate a balanced diet that includes whole grains, lean proteins, fruits, vegetables, and healthy fats. Consult a registered dietitian to create a personalized meal plan.

Regular Exercise: Physical activity is a cornerstone of diabetes management. Find an exercise routine that you enjoy, whether it's walking, swimming, or dancing. Aim for at least 150 minutes of moderate-intensity exercise per week. Remember to monitor your blood sugar before and after exercise.

Medication and Insulin Management: If your treatment plan includes medication or insulin, take them as prescribed by your healthcare provider. Use reminders or apps to ensure you don't miss doses. It's important to understand how your medications work and their potential side effects.

Blood Sugar Monitoring: Regularly monitor your blood sugar levels as recommended by your healthcare provider. Keep a log of your readings and share them with your medical team. Testing your blood sugar at consistent times each day can help identify trends and adjust your management plan accordingly.

Stress Management: Chronic stress can affect blood sugar levels. Incorporate stress-reduction techniques into your daily routine, such as deep breathing, meditation, or mindfulness practices.

Sleep Hygiene: Aim for a consistent sleep schedule and prioritize good sleep hygiene. A good night's sleep is essential for blood sugar control and overall well-being.

Regular Check-ups: Keep your scheduled appointments with your healthcare team. Regular check-ups are essential for monitoring your diabetes, making any necessary adjustments to your treatment plan, and preventing complications.

Goal Setting: Set specific, achievable goals for your diabetes management. This can help you stay motivated and track your progress.

Self-Care: Incorporate self-care activities you enjoy into your routine. This could include hobbies, relaxation time, or spending quality time with loved ones. Taking care of your emotional well-being is as important as physical health.

Adapt to Life Changes: Life is full of changes, and your diabetes management plan may need to adjust accordingly. Adapt to new circumstances, challenges, and experiences as they arise.

Be Patient and Kind to Yourself: Living with diabetes can be demanding, but it's essential to be patient with yourself. If you have setbacks or experience challenges, remember that it's okay, and seeking support is a sign of strength, not weakness.

10.2 Traveling With Diabetes

Whether you travel for business or pleasure, a little extra effort before you leave can make your trip go more smoothly. Just like you plan where you'll stay and check the weather at your destination, you can prep to keep up with your diabetes treatment plan so you'll keep your blood sugar levels in check. Before your trip, tell your doctor about your plans. If you'll be crossing time zones, ask them about how to adjust your insulin doses.

Will you need special meals? Talk to the airline, hotel, or cruise ship about that.

If you're going to visit another country, check to see if you need to get any immunizations before you go. Plan to get them 3 to 4 weeks before your trip. Some shots can affect your blood sugar levels, so ask your doctor about that. And along with learning how to say hello and thank you, learn some diabetes-specific phrases in the local language just in case, such as "I have diabetes" and "I need sugar." You could also scope out health care centers in the places you're going. But remember, if you manage your diabetes well, you shouldn't need to go to one.

Don't forget, your bag should contain medical identification that days you have diabetes, a piece of paper or card with your doctor's name and phone number, a list of all the medicines you take, your prescription drugs, syringes, inhaler and cartridges, and blood sugar testing supplies. Keep them in your carry-on luggage so they don't get lost or sit in an unheated, uncooled cargo hold. Also, enough medicines and diabetes supplies to last an extra week and a quick fix for low blood sugar, like hard candy or juice boxes.

Let your security screener know that you have diabetes and that you've brought medical supplies. You can take them on board, but they must have a prescription label and the maker's label. You can also take syringes with you if you have insulin, too. Do you wear an insulin pump? Tell the security agent. They'll inspect the meter, but ask them not to remove it. When in doubt, check the Transportation Security

Administration website for the latest list of what you can bring with you.

10.2 Diabetes and Relationships

Managing your type 2 diabetes is a big part of your life. If you have a partner or a spouse, diabetes becomes a part of their life, too. Studies show that a supportive partner can help you better manage your disease. And as a bonus, teamwork can bring you closer as a couple. It's obvious but bears saying: No one other than you is more touched by your diabetes than the person who lives with you. Your condition can take an emotional or physical toll on your partner or create conflicts.

It's common for your partner to worry about:

- Serious health complications, like blindness or amputations

- How to help you control your diabetes day to day and to deal with any blood sugar emergencies
- If you'll be able to take care of your family and other responsibilities.
- Money and insurance coverage

If you don't talk about these issues candidly, the stressors over time can put a wedge in your relationship. Here are ways you can strengthen your bond as you navigate your new normal.

Educate Your Partner: The better you understand your diabetes, the better you can manage it. Both of you should learn about the danger of high and low blood sugar levels, insulin and other medications, the benefits of exercise, and the best diet to keep your blood sugar under control.

Consider taking your partner along on your doctors' appointments or to diabetes classes.

Know Your Roles: Every couple is different. You may be grateful if your partner checks that you've taken your insulin or suggests testing new diabetes-friendly recipes. Or you might chafe at those gestures as nagging and controlling. The key is to talk openly and clearly about how to work together so you're as healthy as you can be. Don't assume your loved one will feel burdened by diabetes-related tasks. Also don't expect them to be your caretaker around the clock. Ask them how they'd like to help. Be honest about what support you hope for, too. Clear expectations and boundaries will help you avoid the stress of not enough -- or too much -- support.

Change Together: Managing your diabetes can take a lifestyle overhaul. A healthy diet, regular exercise, and lowering stress are important parts of your medical care. That might mean cooking more often at home or joining a gym. The changes can affect your partner's daily routine in a big way. It's hard to adopt and make new habits stick unless you tackle the challenges as a team. Look for new dishes you both might enjoy, and take up physical activities you can do together, like a 30-minute walk after dinner. You'll both benefit.

Seek Outside Support: If you and your partner feel out of sync in managing your diabetes, couples counseling might help. Whether your diagnosis is new or you've had the condition for a while, a counselor can help you communicate better so your health becomes a shared goal. You could also lean on diabetes support groups. They can help you feel less alone or different and offer advice and tips. Some groups cater to women or men. Others are for couples, families, or even specific ethnic groups. Ask your doctor or diabetes educator about groups near you.

10.4 Parenting With Diabetes

As if parenting wasn't hard enough! When your child or you in particular have diabetes parenting can be even more difficult and require more planning, routine and involvement in your child's life. Children and young people can often rebel against this and it is important to have all carers on the same page to support the child and yourself to feel safe. Parental anxiety is often transferred to the young person so it is important that you have a space to talk away from your child as not every conversation is developmentally appropriate for a child to hear.

Your child is still the young person they were before their diagnosis and can achieve goals, play sports, get a job etc, same as you too as a parent. It is important that there are times at home and while out and about that there is no (or limited) 'Diabetes talk'. Diabetes does not define who they are and this is important to remember. For instance, it is not helpful to say to your child when they first arrive home from school "what is your BGL?"A better question might be 'how was your day at school?"

For you as a parent, first you need to prioritize self-care. Taking care of yourself is essential and ensures you're monitoring your blood sugar level, taking medications or insulin as prescribed, and following a healthy diet and exercise routine. Your well-being directly affects your ability to care for your family. Talk to him too, what diabetes means, how well he could manage his or her diabetes and why it is essential. Most children do not know what this means. You can't blame them because they all just want to enjoy their time as kids, so it's your duty to educate them.

Also, teach by example as a parent you are. Your children learn from your behavior. Use your diabetes management as an opportunity to teach them about the importance of a healthy lifestyle. Involve them in preparing balanced meals and engaging in physical activities together.

10.5 Aging Gracefully With Diabetes

Aging is a natural part of life, and with diabetes, it's essential to adapt your management approach to ensure that you age gracefully while effectively controlling your condition. Embracing a holistic approach to health and well-being is key to enjoying a fulfilling life as you age with diabetes. Here are some tips to help you age gracefully:

Prioritize Diabetes Management: Maintain a proactive approach to diabetes management as you age. Consistently monitor your blood sugar levels, take medications or insulin as prescribed, and follow a balanced diet and exercise routine. Effective management can help prevent diabetes-related complications.

Regular Check-ups: Continue to schedule regular check-ups with your healthcare team. As you age, your health needs may change, so it's crucial to discuss any adjustments needed in your diabetes management plan.

Stay Active: Physical activity is beneficial at any age, and it's especially important as you grow older. Regular exercise can help manage blood sugar, maintain muscle mass, and improve overall health. Consider low-impact exercises like walking, swimming, or yoga to stay active.

Embrace a Healthy Diet: A balanced diet remains essential. As you age, your nutritional needs may evolve, so consult with a registered dietitian to create a meal plan that aligns with your current health status and diabetes management goals.

Manage Your Weight: Maintaining a healthy weight is crucial for diabetes management and overall well-being. As you age, focus on sustainable weight management through a combination of diet and exercise.

Medication and Insulin: If you're taking medications or insulin, follow your treatment plan diligently. Talk to your healthcare provider if you experience any changes in your medication needs as you age.

Heart Health: Pay attention to cardiovascular health. Diabetes can increase the risk of heart disease. Manage your blood pressure and cholesterol levels and incorporate heart-healthy habits into your daily routine.

Bone Health: As you age, consider bone health, especially if you have diabetes. Adequate calcium and vitamin D intake, along with weight-bearing exercises, can help maintain strong bones.

Eye Health: Regular eye check-ups are essential to monitor for diabetes-related eye complications. Age-related eye conditions are also common, so early detection is vital.

Foot Care: Maintain proper foot care to prevent diabetes-related complications. Regularly inspect your feet, moisturize them, and wear comfortable shoes.

Stay Social: Maintain an active social life. Staying connected with friends and family can provide emotional support and contribute to overall well-being.

Stress Management: Adopt stress-reduction techniques, such as meditation, mindfulness, or relaxation exercises. Chronic stress can affect blood sugar levels, and managing it is essential for aging gracefully.

Prioritize Mental Health: Consider your mental health. Aging can bring unique emotional challenges. Seek support from mental health professionals if needed.

Celebrate Achievements: Celebrate your accomplishments and milestones. As you age with diabetes, acknowledge the efforts you've made to maintain your health.

Stay Informed: Stay informed about the latest advancements in diabetes management and treatments. Knowledge is a valuable tool for aging gracefully with diabetes.

Embrace a Positive Attitude: Maintain a positive outlook on life. A positive attitude can help you face the challenges of aging and diabetes with resilience and grace.

Chapter 11: Emerging Therapies and Future of Diabetes Management

11.1 Innovations in Diabetes Care

In recent years, the field of diabetes care has seen remarkable innovations that have transformed the way individuals manage their condition and improve their quality of life. These innovations encompass a wide range of technologies, treatments, and approaches designed to make diabetes management more effective, convenient, and patient-centered.

Continuous Glucose Monitoring (CGM):Continuous Glucose Monitoring has become a game-changer in diabetes management. This device provides real time data on blood glucose levels, helps individuals make decisions concerning dosages, diets and exercises. Some CGMs can predict low or high glucose levels before they occur, enabling proactive interventions.

Insulin Pumps with Automated Insulin Delivery: Insulin pumps have evolved to include automated features that adjust insulin delivery based on CGM data. These closed-loop systems, often referred to as artificial pancreases, can significantly improve blood sugar control while reducing the burden of manual insulin calculations.

Telemedicine and Remote Monitoring: This allows individuals consult healthcare specialists from the comfort of their homes. This helps to minimize frequent in person visit.

Smart Insulin Pens: These apps help users monitor insulin administration, set reminders, and analyze trends in blood glucose levels through their integrated Bluetooth technology. This Bluetooth technology allows user track and transmit dosage data to mobile apps.

Personalized Diabetes Management Apps: These apps have proliferated, offering features like meal planning, glucose tracking, medication reminders, and real-time coaching

Artificial Intelligence (AI): are being used to predict glucose trends and also analyze CGM data.

Advanced Insulin Formulations: New insulin formulations with longer durations of action or faster onset times are being developed. These formulations can provide more flexibility in managing insulin doses and timing.

Closed-Loop Systems for Type 2 Diabetes: Some times ago, these systems were primarily designed for type 1 diabetes. They are used to offer better glucose control and reduce the complexity of diabetes management.

Wearable Devices: Wearable devices, including smartwatches and fitness trackers, are integrating diabetes management features. Some can display glucose levels, provide alerts, and track physical activity.

Artificial Pancreas Implants: Research into fully implantable artificial pancreas devices is ongoing. These devices would eliminate the need for external pumps or sensors.

Bariatric Surgery for Diabetes Management: For individuals with obesity and type 2 diabetes, bariatric surgery has become a more accepted treatment option. It can lead to substantial weight loss and improved blood sugar control.

11.2 Clinical Trials and Research

Clinical trials are part of clinical research and at the heart of all medical advances. It looks at new ways to prevent, detect or treat disease. Scientists are conducting research to learn more about diabetes.

A research is ongoing following more than 5,000 people across the country who have type 2 diabetes to find out which combination of two diabetes medicines is best for blood glucose, also called blood sugar management; has the fewest side effects; and is the most helpful for overall health in long-term diabetes treatment.

Also, other research is being conducted including risk screening for relatives of people with type 1 diabetes, monitoring for people at risk, and innovative clinical trials aimed at slowing down or stopping the disease.

Researchers also use these researches to look at other aspects of care, such as improving the quality of life for people with chronic illnesses.

11.3 Future Possibilities

Diabetes is the major cause of blindness, kidney failure, heart attack, and stroke. It is estimated that the number of people affected by diabetes will rise to 700 million by 2045. This has led the World Health Organization to consider diabetes an epidemic. Despite its huge impact on the global population, there is still no cure for any type of diabetes. Most treatments help patients manage the symptoms to a certain extent, but diabetics still face multiple long-term health complications.

Diabetes affects the regulation of insulin, a hormone required for glucose uptake in cells, resulting in high levels of blood sugar. While there are some similarities in symptoms, the two main types of diabetes develop in different ways. Type 1 diabetes is an autoimmune disease that destroys insulin-producing beta-pancreatic cells. In contrast, patients with type 2 diabetes develop insulin resistance, meaning that insulin is less and less effective at reducing blood sugar. A biotech industry is striving to develop new diabetes treatments and chasing the holy grail: a cure. Let's have a look at what's brewing in the field and how it will change the way diabetes is treated.

For type 1 diabetes, missing cells will be replaced with cell therapy. Although still in the very early stages of development, cell therapy is one of the biggest hopes towards developing a cure for diabetes, especially for type 1 diabetes. Replacing the missing insulin-producing cells could potentially recover normal insulin production and cure patients. However, early attempts to transplant pancreatic cells have largely failed, mostly due to immune reactions that reject and destroy the implanted cells. The lack of donors is also a limitation. One of the most advanced alternatives comes from the

Diabetes Research Institute in the US, which is developing a bioengineered mini-organ where insulin-producing cells are encapsulated within a protective barrier. This mini-pancreas is then implanted into the omentum, a part of the abdominal lining. A phase I/II trial is ongoing, but the DRI announced its first successful results in 2016, revealing that the first patient in Europe treated with this approach no longer requires insulin therapy.

For type 2 diabetes, one of the biggest hits in type 2 diabetes treatment are glucagon-like peptide (GLP)-1 receptor agonists, which induce insulin production in beta-pancreatic cells while suppressing the secretion of glucagon, a hormone with the opposite effect to insulin.

11.4 Diabetes Advocacy

Diabetes is a growing epidemic that cannot be ignored, so when bills are introduced on the federal or state level that positively affect people with diabetes, we are among the first to show support and fight for your rights. And we won't back down until everyone affected by diabetes has the medication and insulin they need to live, until everyone is treated fairly in schools and the workplace regardless of diabetes status, and until health equity is the standard in Congress and in every health care provider's office. Many Americans don't even have access to adequate health care, and we believe health equity is a human right. Our goal is to make insulin affordable and accessible for all who need it, promote health equity for at-risk populations affected by diabetes and prediabetes, put an end to all forms of diabetes discrimination and increase overall funding dedicated to diabetes research and programs.

Away from this book. If you could create time to provide a review if you thought it was worthwhile, it will really motivate me. Thanks in advance.